97 All Natural Meal and Juice Recipes to Treat Urinary Tract Infections:

The Natural Solution to Urinary Tract Infections

By

Joe Correa CSN

COPYRIGHT

This publication is designed to provide accurate and authoritative information in regard to the subject matter covered. It is sold with the understanding that neither the author nor the publisher is engaged in rendering medical advice. If medical advice or assistance is needed, consult with a doctor. This book is considered a guide and should not be used in any way detrimental to your health. Consult with a physician before starting this nutritional plan to make sure it's right for you.

ACKNOWLEDGEMENTS

This book is dedicated to my friends and family that have had mild or serious illnesses so that you may find a solution and make the necessary changes in your life.

97 All Natural Meal and Juice Recipes to Treat Urinary Tract Infections:

The Natural Solution to Urinary Tract Infections

By

Joe Correa CSN

CONTENTS

ABOUT THE AUTHOR

After years of Research, I honestly believe in the positive effects that proper nutrition can have over the body and mind. My knowledge and experience has helped me live healthier throughout the years and which I have shared with family and friends. The more you know about eating and drinking healthier, the sooner you will want to change your life and eating habits.

Nutrition is a key part in the process of being healthy and living longer so get started today. The first step is the most important and the most significant.

INTRODUCTION

97 All Natural Meal and Juice Recipes to Treat Urinary Tract Infections: The Natural Solution to Urinary Tract Infections

By Joe Correa CSN

A urinary infection is a group of rather common infections of any part of the urinary tract – kidneys, ureters, bladder, and urethra. These infections are caused by different microbes (mostly bacteria) that overcome the body's ability to defend itself. This condition leads to more frequent urge to urinate followed by a painful and burning sensation and/or strong smelling urine. Studies show that women are more likely to suffer from urinary infections (with the risk of over 50%) at least once in their life with many cases of repeated infections.

Most urinary infections are caused by bacteria Escherichia coli which can be found in the digestive tract and Chlamydia that attacks urethra. In general, everybody can develop some form of urinary infection. However, there are some risk factors that increase the chances of developing repeated urinary infections. These factors include:

- Improper body hygiene

- Diabetes

- Pregnancy

- Urinary catheter

- Blocked urine flow

- Kidney diseases

- Repeated use of antibiotics which affect the natural microflora

- Weakened immune system

Luckily, most urinary infections are easily curable with antibiotics or antimicrobials. In healthy people (with a normal urinary tract) suffering from some form of urinary infection, the treatment takes about 2-3 days. People whose organisms are weakened by some other disease or condition will most likely get more complicated urinary tract infections and their treatment can take between 7-14 days. Pregnant women, older people, and patients suffering from cancer, diabetes, or some other medical problems should be hospitalized until the infection is completely healed.

Having to deal with urinary infections can be quite unpleasant and can disrupt your everyday life and work. Just like with every other health condition, it's better to prevent these infections from happening in the first place.

For this reason, I have created a wonderful collection of juice recipes that will help you heal any urinary infection. Use these recipes to fix your problem naturally and boost your immune system thus preventing infections in the future.

Enjoy them all and try them during different times of the day. Early morning, when you wake up, is the ideal time for one of these juices.

COMMITMENT

In order to improve my condition, I *(your name)*, commit to eating more of these foods on a daily basis and to exercise at least 30 minutes daily:

- Berries (especially blueberries), peaches, cherries, apples, apricots, oranges, lemon juice, grapefruit, tangerines, mandarins, pears, etc.
- Broccoli, spinach, collard greens, sweet potatoes, avocado, artichoke, baby corn, carrots, celery, cauliflower, onions, etc.
- Whole grains, steel-cut oats, oatmeal, quinoa, barley, etc.
- Black beans, red bean beans, garbanzo beans, lentils, etc.
- Nuts and seeds including: walnuts, cashews, flaxseeds, sesame seeds, etc.
- Fish
- 8 – 10 glasses of water

Sign here

X_____

97 ALL NATURAL MEAL AND JUICE RECIPES TO TREAT URINARY TRACT INFECTIONS

JUICES

1.   Raspberry Cranberry Juice

Ingredients:

1 cup of fresh blueberries

1 cup of fresh raspberries

1 cup of fresh cranberries

1 large lemon, peeled

1 cup of watermelon, seeded

1 tbsp of maple syrup

Preparation:

Combine raspberries, cranberries, and blueberries in a large colander. Rinse under cold running water. Drain and set aside.

Peel the lemon and cut lengthwise in half. Set aside.

Cut the watermelon lengthwise. For one cup, you will need about 1 large wedge. Peel and cut into chunks. Remove the seeds and set aside. Reserve the rest of the melon for some other juices.

Now, process berries, lemon and watermelon in a juicer.

Transfer to serving glasses and stir in the maple syrup.

Add some ice cubes before serving.

Enjoy!

Nutrition information per serving: Kcal: 230, Protein: 4.1g, Carbs: 53.1g, Fats: 1.7g

2.   Apple Celery Juice

Ingredients:

1 medium-sized green apple, cored

3-4 large celery stalks

2 large beets, trimmed

3 large carrots, sliced

1 large lemon, peeled

¼ tsp ginger, ground

A handful of fresh kale, torn

Preparation:

Wash the apple and remove the core. Cut into bite-sized pieces and set aside.

Wash the celery stalks and chop into small pieces. Set aside.

Wash the beets and trim off the green parts. Cut into bite-sized pieces and set aside.

Wash the carrots and cut into thick slices. Set aside.

Peel the lemon and cut lengthwise in half. Set aside.

Wash the kale thoroughly and torn with hands. Set aside.

Now, combine apple, celery, kale, beets, carrots, and lemon in a juicer. Process until juiced.

Transfer to serving glasses and stir in the ginger. Add some ice and serve immediately.

Nutrition information per serving: Kcal: 136, Protein: 6.1g, Carbs: 39g, Fats: 1.2g

3.   Radish Melon Juice

Ingredients:

2 medium-sized radishes

1 medium-sized honeydew melon

1 cup of pomegranate seeds

1 cup of watermelon, seeded

1 cup of beets, trimmed

2 tsp maple syrup

Preparation:

Rinse the beets and radishes and trim off the green parts. Chop into small pieces and set aside.

Cut the honeydew melon lengthwise in half. Scoop out the seeds using a spoon. Cut into large wedges and peel them. Now, cut into small chunks and place in a bowl. Set aside.

Cut the top of the pomegranate fruit using a sharp knife. Slice down to each of the white membranes inside of the fruit. Pop the seeds into a measuring cup and set aside.

Cut the watermelon lengthwise. For one cup, you will need about 1 large wedge. Peel and cut into chunks. Remove the seeds and set aside. Reserve the rest of the melon for some other juices.

Now, combine radishes, honeydew melon, pomegranate seeds, watermelon, and beets in a juicer.

Transfer to serving glasses and stir in the maple syrup.

Add some ice and serve.

Nutrition information per serving: Kcal: 167, Protein: 13.1g, Carbs: 45.9g, Fats: 1.5g

4.   Blueberry Apple Juice

Ingredients:

1 cup of blueberries

1 medium-sized apple, cored

1 cup of beets, trimmed

2 small carrots, sliced

1 large lemon, peeled

2 oz water

Preparation:

Rinse the blueberries under cold running water. Drain and set aside.

Wash the apple and remove the core. Cut into small pieces and set aside.

Wash the beets and trim off the green parts. Cut into bite-sized pieces and set aside.

Wash the carrots and cut into thick slices. Set aside.

Peel the lemon and cut lengthwise in half. Set aside.

Now, combine blueberries, apple, beets, carrots, and lemon in a juicer. Process until juiced.

Transfer to serving glasses and stir in the coconut water. Garnish with mint and refrigerate before serving.

Enjoy!

Nutrition information per serving: Kcal: 240, Protein: 5.6g, Carbs: 74.1g, Fats: 1.5g

5.   Lime Cinnamon Juice

Ingredients:

2 large limes, peeled

¼ tsp of cinnamon, ground

3 large oranges, peeled

2 large lemons, peeled

2 tsp agave nectar

2 oz water

Preparation:

Peel the lemons and limes and cut lengthwise in half. Set aside.

Peel the oranges and divide into wedges. Set aside.

Now, combine limes, oranges, and lemons in a juicer.

Transfer to serving glasses and stir in the cinnamon, agave, and water.

Add few ice cubes and serve immediately.

Nutrition information per serving: Kcal: 246, Protein: 6.8g, Carbs: 83.1g, Fats: 1.1g

6.   Celery Leek Juice

Ingredients:

1 cup fresh celery

3 large leeks, chopped

2 cups beet greens, trimmed

1 cup fresh kale, torn

1 large cucumber, sliced

¼ tsp ginger powder

Preparation:

Wash the beet greens and kale thoroughly and torn with hands. Set aside.

Peel the onion and cut in half. Cut one slice and reserve the rest for some other juice or meal.

Wash the celery and leek. Cut into small pieces and set aside.

Wash the cucumber and cut into thick slices. Set aside.

Now, combine celery, leek, beet greens, cucumber, and ginger in a juicer. Process until juiced.

Transfer to serving glasses and refrigerate for 5 minutes before serving.

Nutritional information per serving: Kcal: 230, Protein: 11.5g, Carbs: 63.2g, Fats: 2.1g

7.   Strawberry Apple Juice

Ingredients:

1 cup fresh strawberries, chopped

1 medium-sized Red Delicious apple, cored

1 cup fresh blackberries

1 cup green grapes

2 oz coconut water

Preparation:

Combine strawberries and blackberries in a colander. Wash under cold running water and set aside.

Wash the apple and remove the core. Cut into bite-sized pieces and set aside.

Rinse the grapes and remove the stems. Set aside.

Now, combine strawberries, apple, blackberries, and grapes in a juicer. Process until juiced. Transfer to serving glasses and stir in the coconut water.

Add some ice cubes before serving.

Nutritional information per serving: Kcal: 201, Protein: 4.3g, Carbs: 63.4g, Fats: 1.7g

8.   Cucumber Cantaloupe Juice

Ingredients:

1 large cucumber

1 cup cantaloupe, cubed

1 large honeydew melon wedge

1 cup watermelon, seeded

1 tbsp agave nectar

Preparation:

Wash the cucumber and cut into thick slices. Set aside.

Cut the cantaloupe in half. Scoop out the seeds and flesh. Cut two wedges and peel them. Chop into chunks and set aside. Reserve the rest of the cantaloupe in a refrigerator.

Cut the honeydew melon lengthwise in half. Scoop out the seeds using a spoon. Cut one large wedge and peel. Cut into small chunks and place in a bowl. Wrap the rest of the melon in a plastic foil and refrigerate.

Cut the watermelon lengthwise. For one cup, you will need about 1 large wedge. Peel and cut into chunks. Remove the seeds and set aside. Reserve the rest of for some other juices.

Now, combine cucumber, cantaloupe, honeydew melon, and watermelon in a juicer.

Transfer to serving glasses and stir in the agave. Add some ice before serving.

Enjoy!

Nutritional information per serving: Kcal: 201, Protein: 3.4g, Carbs: 57.6g, Fats: 0.8g

9. Lettuce Watermelon Juice

Ingredients:

2 cups red leaf lettuce, shredded

1 cup watermelon, diced

2 cups raspberries

1 cup beets, chopped

¼ cup water

Preparation:

Wash the lettuce thoroughly and torn with hands. Set aside.

Cut the watermelon lengthwise. For one cup, you will need about 1 large wedge. Peel and cut into chunks. Remove the seeds and set aside. Reserve the rest of for some other juices.

Wash the raspberries under cold running water. Drain and set aside.

Wash the beets and trim off the green parts. Cut into small pieces and set aside.

Now, combine lettuce, watermelon, raspberries, and beets in a juicer.

Transfer to serving glasses and stir in the water.

Add some ice and serve immediately.

Nutritional information per serving: Kcal: 157, Protein: 6.8g, Carbs: 55g, Fats: 2.1g

10.   Orange Chard Juice

Ingredients:

2 large oranges, peeled

1 cup Swiss chard, chopped

4 large cucumbers, peeled

3 large carrots, chopped

Preparation:

Peel the oranges and divide into wedges. Set aside.

Rinse the Swiss chard thoroughly under cold running water using a colander. Roughly chop it and set aside.

Wash the cucumbers and carrots. Cut into thick slices and set aside.

Now, combine oranges, Swiss chard, cucumbers, and carrots in a juicer and process until juiced.

Transfer to serving glasses and add some ice cubes.

Enjoy!

Nutritional information per serving: Kcal: 283, Protein: 9g, Carbs: 88.9g, Fats: 1.6g

11.   Squash Pear Juice

Ingredients:

4 cups butternut squash, sliced

1 large pear, cored

1 cup of purple cabbage, shredded

½ cup water

Preparation:

Peel the butternut squash and cut in half. Scoop out the seeds using a spoon. Cut into small chunks and set aside. Reserve the rest in the refrigerator.

Wash the pear and remove the core. Cut into bite-sized pieces and set aside.

Rinse the cabbage thoroughly and shred it. Set aside.

Now, combine butternut squash, pear, and green cabbage in a juicer and process until juiced.

Transfer to serving glasses and stir in the water.

Add some ice and serve immediately.

Nutritional information per serving: Kcal: 192, Protein: 7g, Carbs: 59.9g, Fats: 1.7g

12.   Avocado Celery Juice

Ingredients:

1 cup avocado, sliced

1 cup celery, chopped

1 tbsp fresh mint, finely chopped

1 cup green cabbage, torn

½ cup coconut water, unsweetened

Preparation:

Peel the avocado and cut in half. Remove the pit and cut into chunks. Set aside.

Wash the celery and cut into small pieces. Set aside.

Wash the cabbage thoroughly and torn with hands. Set aside.

Now, combine avocado, celery, and cabbage in a juicer. Process until juiced. Transfer to serving glasses and stir in coconut water and fresh mint.

Add some ice before serving.

Enjoy!

Nutritional information per serving: Kcal: 219, Protein: 4.8g, Carbs: 20.8g, Fats: 21.6g

13.   Orange Grapefruit Juice

Ingredients:

2 large oranges, peeled

1 large grapefruit, peeled

2 cups asparagus, chopped

1 tbsp mint, finely chopped

¼ cup of water

Preparation:

Peel the oranges and grapefruit. Divide into wedges and set aside.

Rinse the asparagus under cold running water. Trim off the woody ends and chop into small pieces. Fill the measuring cups and set aside.

Now, combine asparagus, oranges, and grapefruit in a juicer and process until juiced.

Transfer to serving glasses and stir in the finely chopped mint and water. Add few ice cubes and serve immediately.

Nutritional information per serving: Kcal: 255, Protein: 11.2g, Carbs: 79.8g, Fats: 1.1g

14.   Granny Smith's Juice

Ingredients:

1 cup pineapple, chopped

1 cup sweet cherries, pitted

1 large Honeycrisp apple, cored

2 large kiwis, peeled

Preparation:

Cut the top of a pineapple and peel it using a sharp knife. Cut into small chunks. Reserve the rest of the pineapple in a refrigerator.

Wash the cherries under cold running water. Drain and remove the pits. Set aside.

Wash the apple and remove the core. Cut into bite-sized pieces and set aside.

Peel the kiwis and cut lengthwise in half. Set aside.

Now, combine pineapple, cherries, apple, and kiwis in a juicer and process until juiced.

Transfer to serving glasses and serve immediately.

Nutrition information per serving: Kcal: 287, Protein: 4.2g, Carbs: 84.5g, Fats: 1.2g

15. Blackberry Banana Juice

Ingredients:

1 cup of blackberries

1 large banana, peeled

1 cup of blueberries

1 tsp maple syrup

½ tsp cinnamon, ground

Preparation:

Combine blackberries and blueberries in a colander. Rinse under cold running water and drain. Set aside.

Peel the banana and chop into chunks. Set aside.

Now, combine berries and banana in a juicer. Process until juiced.

Transfer to serving glasses and stir in the honey and cinnamon.

Add some ice and serve immediately.

Enjoy!

Nutritional information per serving: Kcal: 229, Protein: 4.5g, Carbs: 76.3g, Fats: 1.6g

16. Blackberry Cucumber Juice

Ingredients:

1 cup of fresh blackberries

1 large cucumber, sliced

1 cup pomegranate seeds

1 whole lime, peeled

A handful of fresh parsley

Preparation:

Rinse the blackberries under cold running water. Drain and set aside.

Wash the cucumber and cut into thick slices. Set aside.

Cut the top of the pomegranate fruit using a sharp knife. Slice down to each of the white membranes inside of the fruit. Pop the seeds into a medium bowl.

Peel the lime and cut in half. Set aside.

Rinse the parsley thoroughly and roughly chop with hands. Set aside.

Now, combine pomegranate seeds, blackberries, cucumber, lime, and parsley in a juicer. Process until juiced.

Transfer to serving glasses and add some ice cubes before serving.

Nutritional information per serving: Kcal: 152, Protein: 8.1g, Carbs: 58.6g, Fats: 2.7g

17.   Parsnip Celery Juice

1 cup parsnips, chopped

1 large celery stalk, chopped

1 whole guava, chopped

2 large grapefruits, peeled

¼ cup water

Preparation:

Wash the parsnips and cut into small slices. Set aside.

Rinse the celery and cut into small pieces. Set aside.

Wash the guava and cut into chunks. If you are using large fruit, reserve the rest for some other recipe in a refrigerator.

Peel the grapefruits and chop into bite-sized pieces.

Now, combine parsnips, celery, guava, grapefruits in a juicer. Process until juiced.

Transfer to serving glasses and add some ice before serving.

Nutritional information per serving: Kcal: 279, Protein: 7.2g, Carbs: 86g, Fats: 1.7g

18.   Apple Goji Juice

Ingredients:

2 small Granny Smith's apples, cored

1 cup goji berries

1 cup fresh cherries, pitted

1 cup beets

3 large tomatoes, peeled

Preparation:

Wash the apples and remove the core. Cut into bite-sized pieces and set aside.

Place the goji berries in a medium bowl and add 1 cup of hot water. Soak for 10 minutes before juicing. Remove the water and set aside.

Wash the beets and trim off the green parts. Cut into small pieces and set aside.

Wash the cherries and remove the pits. Set aside.

Rinse the tomatoes and place in a bowl. Chop into quarters and reserve the juice while cutting.

Now, combine apples, goji berries, beets, cherries, and tomatoes in a juicer.

Transfer to serving glasses and stir in the reserved tomato juice.

Refrigerate for 10 minutes before serving.

Nutritional information per serving: Kcal: 318, Protein: 9.5g, Carbs: 98g, Fats: 2.4g

19.　Cranberry Pineapple Juice

Ingredients:

1 cup cranberries

1 cup pineapple, chunked

1 medium-sized apple, chopped

1 cup apricot, sliced

¼ cup water

Preparation:

Rinse the cranberries under cold running water using a large colander. Drain and fill the measuring cup. Reserve the rest for later.

Cut the top and peel the pineapple. Chop into small chunks and fill the measuring cup. Reserve the rest in the refrigerator for some other juice.

Wash the apple and cut in half. Remove the core and cut into bite-sized pieces. Set aside.

Wash the apricot and cut in half. Remove the pit and chop into small pieces. Set aside.

Now, combine cranberries, pineapple, apple, and apricot in a juicer. Process until well juiced. Transfer to serving glasses and stir in the water.

Serve immediately.

Nutrition information per serving: Kcal: 248, Protein: 4.3g, Carbs: 76.1g, Fats: 1.3g

20.   Cucumber Maple Juice

Ingredients:

1 medium-sized cucumber, sliced

2 tsp maple syrup

1 cup strawberries, chopped

1 cup spinach, torn

2 oz water

Preparation:

Wash the cucumber and cut into thin slices.

Wash the strawberries and remove the stems. Cut into bite-sized pieces and set aside.

Wash the spinach thoroughly under cold running water. Slightly drain and torn into small pieces. Set aside.

Now, combine cucumber, strawberries, and spinach in a juicer and process until juiced. Transfer to a serving glass and stir in the water and maple syrup.

Refrigerate for 5 minutes before serving.

Enjoy!

Nutrition information per serving: Kcal: 83, Protein: 6.9g, Carbs: 24.6g, Fats: 1.3g

21.   Blackberry Plum Juice

Ingredients:

1 cup fresh blackberries

1 cup plums, halved

1 cup turnip greens, chopped

½ tsp ginger, ground

1 tsp agave nectar

½ cup water

Preparation:

Wash the blackberries under cold running water. Set aside.

Wash the plums and cut in half. Remove the pits and set aside.

Rinse the turnip greens and torn with hands. Set aside.

Now, combine blackberries, plums, and turnip greens in a juicer. Process until juiced. Transfer to a serving glass and stir in the agave, ginger, and water.

Refrigerate for 5 minutes before serving.

Enjoy!

Nutrition information per serving: Kcal: 141, Protein: 4.2g, Carbs: 40.3g, Fats: 1.4g

22.   Cranberry Leek Juice

Ingredients:

1 cup fresh cranberries

1 cup leek, chopped

2 cups cherries, pitted

2 tbsp fresh mint, finely chopped

¼ cup coconut water

Preparation:

Rinse the cranberries and cherries under cold running water using a colander. Drain and set aside.

Rinse the leek and chop into small pieces. Set aside.

Cut the cherries into halves. Remove the pits and set aside.

Combine cranberries, leek, cherries, and mint in a juicer and process until juiced. Transfer to serving glasses and stir in the coconut water.

Add some ice and serve!

Nutrition information per serving: Kcal: 252, Protein: 5.3g, Carbs: 79.5g, Fats: 1.8g

23. Peach Lettuce Juice

Ingredients:

1 large peach, chopped

1 cup of Iceberg lettuce, torn

2 large Red Delicious apples

1 large carrot, sliced

½ cup coconut water

½ lemon, peeled

Preparation:

Wash the peach and cut in half. Remove the pit and chop into small pieces. Set aside.

Rinse the lettuce thoroughly and torn with hands. Set aside.

Wash the apples and cut in half. Remove the core and cut into bite-sized pieces. Set aside.

Wash the carrot and cut into thick slices. Set aside.

Peel the lemon and cut lengthwise in half. Reserve the rest for later.

Now, combine peach, lettuce, apples, carrot, and lemon in a juicer and process until juiced.

Transfer to serving glasses and refrigerate for 5 minutes before serving.

Nutrition information per serving: Kcal: 263, Protein: 5.1g, Carbs: 84.5g, Fats: 1.2g

24.   Green Kiwi Apple Juice

Ingredients:

2 large kiwis, peeled

1 medium-sized Honeycrisp apple, cored

1 cup of fresh spinach

1 large cucumber, sliced

¼ tsp ginger powder

Preparation:

Peel the kiwis and cut lengthwise in half. Set aside.

Wash the apple and remove the core. Cut into bite-sized pieces and set aside.

Wash the spinach thoroughly and torn with hands. Place in a pot of boiling water and let it soak for 5 minutes, or until wilted. Set aside.

Wash the cucumber and cut into thick slices. Set aside.

Peel the ginger root slice and set aside.

Combine kiwis, apple, cucumber, and soaked spinach in a juicer. Process until well juiced. Transfer to a serving glass and add some ice before serving.

Nutrition information per serving: Kcal: 201, Protein: 13.2g, Carbs: 56.5g, Fats: 2.6g

25.   Melon Agave Juice

Ingredients:

1 cup of watermelon, seeded

2 tsp agave nectar

1 cup blueberries

1 cup raspberries

1 cup cranberries

1 whole lime, peeled

Preparation:

Cut the watermelon lengthwise. Cut one large wedge. Peel and cut into chunks. Remove the seeds and set aside. Reserve the rest of the melon in the refrigerator

Combine blueberries, raspberries, and cranberries in a colander and rinse under cold running water. Drain and set aside.

Peel the lime and cut lengthwise in half. Set aside.

Now, combine watermelon, blueberries, raspberries, cranberries, and lemon in a juicer. Process until juiced. Transfer to serving glasses and stir in the agave nectar.

Add some ice cubes before serving.

Enjoy!

Nutrition information per serving: Kcal: 229, Protein: 4.1g, Carbs: 54.3g, Fats: 1.6g

26.   Cherry Apple Juice

Ingredients:

1 cup fresh cherries, pitted

2 large red apples, cored

1 large banana, chopped

1 cup watercress

A handful of fresh spinach

Preparation:

Rinse the cherries under cold running water. Drain and cut in half. Remove the pits and set aside.

Wash the apple and cut in half. Remove the core and chop into small pieces. Set aside.

Peel the banana and cut into small chunks. Set aside.

Combine watercress and spinach in a colander and wash thoroughly. Torn with hands and set aside.

Now, combine cherries, apples, banana, watercress, and spinach in a juicer and process until juiced.

Transfer to serving glasses and add few ice cubes before serving.

Enjoy!

Nutrition information per serving: Kcal: 390, Protein: 6.6g, Carbs: 113g, Fats: 1.7g

27.   Grape Pear Juice

Ingredients:

1 cup green grapes

1 large pear, cored

1 medium-sized lemon, peeled

2 large cucumbers, sliced

Preparation:

Rinse the green grapes under cold running water. Drain and remove the stems. Fill the measuring cup and set aside.

Rinse the pear and remove the core. Cut into bite-sized pieces and set aside.

Peel the lemon and cut into quarters. Set aside.

Wash the cucumbers and cut into thin slices. Set aside.

Now, combine grapes, pear, lemon, and cucumber in a juicer. Process until juiced. Transfer to serving glasses and stir well.

Refrigerate for 5-10 minutes before serving.

Enjoy!

Nutrition information per serving: Kcal: 119, Protein: 18.6g, Carbs: 32.2g, Fats: 0.2g

28.   Lime Carrot Juice

Ingredients:

3 large carrots, sliced

1 large lime, peeled

½ cup cucumber, sliced

1 large pear, cored

¼ cup fresh mint

½ cup broccoli, chopped

¼ tsp ginger powder

2 oz water

Preparation:

Wash and peel the carrots. Remove the tops and cut into thin slices.

Peel the lime and cut into quarters. Set aside.

Peel the cucumber and chop into small pieces. Fill the measuring cup and reserve the rest in the refrigerator. Set aside.

Wash the pear and remove the core. Cut into bite-sized pieces and set aside.

Combine broccoli and mint in a large colander. Rinse under cold running water. Drain and set aside.

Now, combine carrots, lime, cucumber, pear, mint, broccoli, and ginger powder in a juicer. Process until juiced.

Transfer to serving glasses and stir in the water

Refrigerate for 10 minutes before serving.

Nutrition information per serving: Kcal: 141, Protein: 5.5g, Carbs: 45.7g, Fats: 0.9g

29.   Carrot Fuji Juice

Ingredients:

1 cup fresh strawberries, chopped

1 large carrot, sliced

1 medium-sized Fuji apple, cored and chopped

1 medium-sized orange, peeled and wedged

1 cup cucumber, sliced

Preparation:

Wash the carrot and cut into thin slices. Set aside.

Wash the apple and cut in half. Remove the core and cut into bite-sized pieces. Set aside.

Wash the strawberries and remove the top stems. Cut into small pieces and set aside.

Peel the orange and divide into wedges. Set aside.

Wash the cucumber and cut into thin slices. Set aside.

Combine carrots, apple, strawberries, orange, and cucumber in a juicer. Process until juiced. Transfer to the serving glasses refrigerate for 5-10 minutes before serving.

Enjoy!

Nutrition information per serving: Kcal: 104, Protein: 3.9g, Carbs: 31.2g, Fats: 1.1g

30.   Apple Vanilla Juice

Ingredients:

1 large Granny Smith's apple, cored and chopped

1 large lemon, peeled

1 large cucumber, sliced

¼ tsp vanilla extract

Preparation:

Wash the apple and remove the core. Cut into bite-sized pieces and set aside.

Peel the lemon and cut into quarters. Set aside.

Wash the cucumber and cut into thick slices. Set aside.

Wash the fresh mint and soak in water for 5 minutes.

Now, combine apple, lemon, cucumber, and mint in a juicer and process until juiced.

Transfer to serving glasses and stir in the peppermint extract.

Garnish with some extra mint leaves and add some ice before serving.

Enjoy!

Nutrition information per serving: Kcal: 170, Protein: 2.3g, Carbs: 22.3g, Fats: 1.4g

31.   Kiwi Watermelon Juice

Ingredients:

1 large kiwi, peeled

2 cups watermelon, chopped

1 cup raspberries

1 large orange, peeled

2 oz coconut water

Preparation:

Peel the kiwi and cut lengthwise in half. Set aside.

Cut the watermelon lengthwise. For two cups, you will need about two large wedges. Peel and cut into chunks. Remove the seeds and set aside. Reserve the rest of the melon for some other juices. Set aside.

Rinse the raspberries thoroughly under cold running water. Drain and set aside.

Peel the orange and divide into wedges. Set aside.

Now, combine kiwi, watermelon, raspberries, and orange in a juicer. Process until juiced and transfer to serving glasses. Stir in the coconut water and refrigerate for a while before serving.

Enjoy!

Nutrition information per serving: Kcal: 232, Protein: 5.8g, Carbs: 71.4g, Fats: 1.8g

32.   Pineapple Mint Juice

Ingredients:

1 cup pineapple, chopped

1 tbsp fresh mint, chopped

2 large limes, peeled

1 cup guava, chopped

1 large cucumber, sliced

Preparation:

Peel the limes and cut lengthwise in half. Set aside.

Wash the guava and cut into bite-sized pieces. Fill the measuring cup and reserve the rest for some other recipe in a refrigerator.

Cut the top of a pineapple and peel it using a sharp knife. Cut into bite-sized pieces and fill the measuring cup. Reserve the rest of the pineapple in a refrigerator.

Wash the cucumber and cut into thin slices. Set aside.

Place chopped mint into a small bowl and add 3 tbsp of boiling water. Let it sit for 5 minutes.

Now, combine pineapple, limes, guava, and cucumber in a juicer. Process until well juiced and transfer to serving glasses. Drain the mint water and add to juice. Refrigerate for 10-15 minutes before serving.

Nutrition information per serving: Kcal: 158, Protein: 4.7g, Carbs: 47.9g, Fats: 1.1g

33. Cucumber Plum Juice

Ingredients:

1 large cucumber, sliced

5 whole plums, pitted

1 cup blackberries

3 small strawberries, chopped

1 cup Romaine lettuce, chopped

2 oz water

Preparation:

Wash the cucumber and cut into thin slices. Set aside.

Wash the plums and cut in half. Remove the pits and cut into quarters. Set aside.

Wash the blackberries under cold running water using a colander. Slightly drain and set aside.

Wash the strawberries and remove the stems. Cut into halves and set aside.

Rinse the lettuce thoroughly under cold running water. Drain and roughly chop it. Set aside.

Now, combine cucumber, plums, blackberries, strawberries, and lettuce in a juicer and process until juice. Transfer to serving glasses and stir in the water.

Refrigerate for 10 minutes before serving.

Nutrition information per serving: Kcal: 221, Protein: 7.5g, Carbs: 69.1g, Fats: 2.1g

34.   Pomegranate Carrot Juice

Ingredients:

1 cup pomegranate seeds

1 large carrot, peeled

1 large lemon, peeled

1 large apricot, pitted

1 large orange, wedged

2 oz coconut water

Preparation:

Cut the top of the pomegranate fruit using a sharp knife. Slice down to each of the white membranes inside of the fruit. Pop the seeds into measuring cup and set aside.

Peel and wash the carrot. Cut into thin slices and set aside.

Peel the lemon and cut lengthwise in half. Set aside.

Wash the apricot and cut in half. Remove the pit and cut into small pieces. Set aside.

Peel the orange and divide into wedges. Set aside.

Combine pomegranate seeds, carrot, lemon, apricot, and orange in a juicer. Process until well juiced and transfer to serving glasses. Stir in the coconut water and add few ice cubes before serving.

Nutrition information per serving: Kcal: 241, Protein: 7.3g, Carbs: 73.9g, Fats: 2.3g

35.   Peach Kiwi Juice

Ingredients:

2 large peaches, pitted

1 large kiwi, peeled

1 large Fuji apple, cored and chopped

1 large orange, peeled

1 cup strawberries, chopped

1 large lemon, peeled

2 oz water

Preparation:

Wash the peaches and cut in half. Remove the pits and cut into small pieces. Set aside.

Peel the kiwi and lemon. Cut lengthwise into halves and set aside.

Wash the apple and cut in half. Remove the core and cut into bite-sized pieces. Set aside.

Peel the orange and divide into wedges. Cut each wedge in half and set aside.

Wash the strawberries under cold running water. Remove the green parts and cut into bite-sized pieces. Set aside.

Combine peaches, kiwi, lemon, apple, orange, and strawberries in a juicer. Process until well juiced. Transfer to serving glasses and stir in the water. Add some ice and serve.

Enjoy!

Nutrition information per serving: Kcal: 345, Protein: 7.8g, Carbs: 105g, Fats: 2.3g

36.   Pomegranate Apple Juice

Ingredients:

1 cup of pomegranate seeds

1 large green apple, cored

1 cup cranberries

4 whole plums, pitted and chopped

1 tsp maple syrup

Preparation:

Cut the top of the pomegranate fruit using a sharp knife. Slice down to each of the white membranes inside of the fruit. Pop the seeds into a measuring cup and set aside.

Wash the apple and cut in half. Remove the core and cut into bite-sized pieces. Set aside.

Wash the cranberries thoroughly and drain. Set aside.

Wash the plums and cut in half. Remove the pits and cut into bite-sized pieces. Set aside.

Now, combine pomegranate, apple, cranberries, and plums in a juicer. Process until well juiced. Transfer to a serving glass and stir in the maple syrup. Optionally, add some ice before serving.

Enjoy!

Nutrition information per serving: Kcal: 264, Protein: 4.5g, Carbs: 78.6g, Fats: 1.1g

37.   Sour Spinach Lemon Juice

Ingredients:

1 cup fresh spinach, chopped

1 whole lemon, peeled

1 cup cranberries

1 cup beet greens, chopped

½ cup water

Preparation:

Wash the baby spinach thoroughly and torn it with hands.

Peel the lemon and cut lengthwise. Set aside.

Place the cranberries in a colander and wash under cold running water. Drain and set aside.

Rinse the beet greens under running water using a colander. Roughly chop it using hands and set aside.

Combine spinach, lemon, cranberries, and turnip greens in a juicer. Process until juiced. Transfer to serving glasses and stir in the water.

Add some ice and serve immediately.

Nutritional information per serving: Kcal: 51, Protein: 4.3g, Carbs: 23.6g, Fats: 0.4g

38.   Sweet Strawberry Juice

Ingredients:

1 cup of strawberries, chopped

1 large Granny Smith's apple, cored

1 cup cranberries

1 large carrot, sliced

1 whole lemon, peeled

1 large orange, peeled and wedged

1 tsp stevia powder

Preparation:

Place the strawberries and cranberries in a colander and wash under cold running water. Drain and cut in half. Set aside.

Wash the apple and remove the core. Cut into bite-sized pieces and set aside.

Wash the carrot and cut into thick slices. Set aside.

Peel the lemon cut lengthwise in half. Set aside.

Peel the orange and divide into wedges. Set aside.

Combine apple, cranberries, strawberries, carrots, lemon, and orange in juicer and process until juiced. Transfer to serving glasses and stir in the water and stevia powder.

Add few ice cubes, or refrigerate for a while minutes before serving.

Nutritional information per serving: Kcal: 268, Protein: 5.6g, Carbs: 89.1g, Fats: 1.6g

39.   Squash Orange Juice

Ingredients:

2 cups butternut squash, chopped

1 large orange, peeled and wedged

1 cup pomegranate seeds

1 whole lemon, peeled

1 cup celery, chopped

2 oz water

Preparation:

Peel the butternut squash and remove the seeds using a spoon. Cut into small cubes and reserve the rest of the squash for some other recipe. Wrap in a plastic foil and refrigerate.

Peel the orange and lemon. Divide orange into wedges and cut lemon lengthwise in half. Set aside.

Wash the celery and chop into small pieces. Set aside.

Cut the top of the pomegranate fruit using a sharp knife. Slice down to each of the white membranes inside of the fruit. Pop the seeds into a medium bowl.

Now, combine butternut squash, orange, pomegranate seeds, lemon, and celery in a juicer and process until juiced.

Transfer to serving glasses and stir in the water. Add few ice cubes and serve.

Enjoy!

Nutritional information per serving: Kcal: 251, Protein: 7.3g, Carbs: 79g, Fats: 1.8g

40.   Grapefruit Cucumber Juice

Ingredients:

1 large grapefruit, peeled and wedged

1 large cucumber, sliced

1 cup papaya, chopped

1 small Red Delicious apple, cored and chopped

2 oz coconut water

1 tsp maple syrup

Preparation:

Peel the grapefruit and divide into wedges. Set aside.

Wash the cucumber and cut into thick slices. Set aside.

Peel the papaya and cut lengthwise in half. Scoop out the black seeds and flesh using a spoon. Cut into small chunks and fill the measuring cup. Reserve the rest for some other juice. Set aside.

Wash the apple and remove the core. Cut into bite-sized pieces and set aside.

Combine grapefruit, cucumber, papaya, and apple in a juicer. Transfer to serving glasses and stir in the coconut water and maple syrup.

Add few ice cubes and serve immediately.

Nutritional information per serving: Kcal: 264, Protein: 5.1g, Carbs: 76.9g, Fats: 1.3g

41. Fuji Orange Juice

Ingredients:

1 small Fuji apple, cored

1 large carrot, sliced

1 large orange, peeled and wedged

1 cup cherries, halved and pitted

1 whole lemon, peeled

2 oz water

Preparation:

Wash the apple and remove the core. Cut into bite-sized pieces and set aside.

Peel the orange and lemon. Divide orange into wedges and cut lemon lengthwise in half. Set aside.

Wash the carrot and cut into thick slices. Set aside.

Wash the cherries thoroughly and cut into halves. Remove the pits and set aside.

Now, combine apple, orange, carrot, lemon, cherries in a juicer and process until juiced. Transfer to serving glasses and add some ice before serving.

Enjoy!

Nutritional information per serving: Kcal: 253, Protein: 5.3g, Carbs: 78.2g, Fats: 1.1g

42. Kiwi Maple Juice

Ingredients:

2 large kiwis, peeled

1 large lemon, peeled

1 cup pineapple, chunked

1 large carrot, sliced

1 large yellow apple, cored

1 tsp maple syrup

Preparation:

Peel the kiwis and lemon. Cut lengthwise into halves and set aside.

Cut the top of a pineapple and peel it using a sharp knife. Cut into small chunks and fill the measuring cup. Reserve the rest of the pineapple in a refrigerator.

Wash the carrot and cut into thick slices. Set aside.

Wash the apple and remove the core. Cut into bite-sized pieces and set aside.

Now, combine kiwis, lemon, pineapple, carrot, and apple in a juicer. Transfer to serving glasses and stir in the maple syrup. Optionally, add some ice before serving.

Nutritional information per serving: Kcal: 132, Protein: 8.9g, Carbs: 35.4g, Fats: 1.7g

43.   Coconut Watermelon Juice

Ingredients:

1 cup watermelon, seeded and chopped

1 cup mango, chopped

1 large Granny Smith's apple, cored

1 cup black grapes, stems removed

2 oz fresh coconut water

Preparation:

Cut the watermelon lengthwise. For one cup, you will need about 1 large wedge. Peel and cut into chunks. Remove the seeds and set aside. Reserve the rest for some other juice.

Wash the mango and cut into chunks. Set aside.

Wash the apple and remove the core. Cut into bite-sized pieces and set aside.

Wash the green grapes using a colander and set aside.

Now, combine grapes, watermelon, mango, and apple in a juicer and process until juiced.

Transfer to serving glasses and stir in the coconut water. Add few ice cubes or refrigerate before serving.

Enjoy!

Nutritional information per serving: Kcal: 288, Protein: 3.7g, Carbs: 80g, Fats: 1.5g

44.   Sour Cherry Grape Juice

Ingredients:

1 cup sour cherries, pitted

2 cups green grapes

1 small banana, peeled

1 whole lime, peeled

1 tbsp coconut water

Preparation:

Rinse the cherries using a colander. Drain and cut each in half. Remove the pits and fill the measuring cup. Reserve the rest in the refrigerator.

Rinse the grapes under cold running water and remove the stems. Set aside.

Peel the banana and cut into chunks. Set aside.

Peel the lime and cut lengthwise in half. Set aside.

Now, combine cherries, grapes, banana, and lime in a juicer and process until juiced. Transfer to a serving glass and stir in the coconut water.

Serve immediately.

Nutrition information per serving: Kcal: 292, Protein: 4.1g, Carbs: 82.9g, Fats: 1.3g

45.　　Cucumber Pomegranate Juice

Ingredients:

1 cup cucumber, sliced

½ cup pomegranate seeds

1 cup pumpkin, cubed

1 whole lemon, peeled

1 cup broccoli, chopped

Preparation:

Wash the cucumber and cut into thin slices. Fill the measuring cup and reserve the rest in the refrigerator. Set aside.

Cut the top of the pomegranate fruit using a sharp knife. Slice down to each of the white membranes inside of the fruit. Pop the seeds into a measuring cup and reserve the rest in the refrigerator for some other recipe.

Cut the top of a pumpkin. Cut lengthwise in half and then scrape out the seeds. Cut one large wedge and peel it. Cut into small cubes and fill the measuring cup. Reserve the rest in the refrigerator.

Peel the lemon and cut lengthwise in half. Set aside.

Wash the broccoli and trim off the outer leaves. Cut into bite-sized pieces and fill the measuring cup. Reserve the rest for later.

Trim off the outer wilted layers of the fennel. Roughly chop it and fill the measuring cup. Reserve the rest for later.

Now, combine cucumber, pomegranate seeds, pumpkin, lemon, and broccoli in a juicer and process until well juiced. Transfer to a serving glass and optionally, add some honey or agave nectar for a sweet taste.

Add some crushed ice and serve.

Nutrition information per serving: Kcal: 210, Protein: 3.9g, Carbs: 63.7g, Fats: 2.3g

46.   Mango Mint Juice

Ingredients:

1 cup mango, chunked

1 cup fresh mint, torn

1 small Golden Delicious apple, cored

1 medium-sized peach, pitted

2 medium-sized strawberries, chopped

Preparation:

Peel the mango and cut into small chunks. Fill the measuring cup and reserve the rest in the refrigerator.

Rinse the mint thoroughly under cold running water and torn with hands. Set aside. You can soak mint in hot water for 2 minutes, but it's optional.

Wash the apple and cut lengthwise in half. Remove the core and cut into bite-sized pieces. Set aside.

Wash the peach and cut in half. Remove the pit and cut into small pieces. Set aside.

Wash the strawberries and remove the stems. Cut into small pieces and set aside.

Now, combine mint, apple, mango, peach, and strawberries in a juicer and process until well juiced. Transfer to a serving glass and add few ice cubes.

Serve immediately.

Nutrition information per serving: Kcal: 227, Protein: 4.1g, Carbs: 64.9g, Fats: 1.6g

47.   Cranberry Sage Juice

Ingredients:

1 cup cranberries

1 cup cucumber, sliced

1 large honeydew melon wedge

2 large strawberries, chopped

1 oz coconut water

2 tsp fresh sage, finely chopped

Preparation:

Wash the cucumber and cut into thin slices. Fill the measuring cup and reserve the rest for later. Set aside.

Using a small colander, rinse well the cranberries. Drain and set aside.

Cut melon lengthwise in half. Scoop out the seeds and then wash the melon. Cut one wedge and peel it. Cut into bite-sized pieces and set aside.

Wash the strawberries and remove the stems. Chop into small pieces and set aside.

Now, combine cranberries, cucumber melon, and strawberries in a juicer. Process until well juiced. Transfer to a serving glass and stir in the coconut water and sage.

Serve immediately.

Nutrition information per serving: Kcal: 96, Protein: 1.8g, Carbs: 31.4g, Fats: 0.6g

48.　　Banana Plum Juice

Ingredients:

1 cup banana, chunked

2 whole plums, chopped

1 cup strawberries, chopped

1 cup cantaloupe, chopped

¼ tsp cinnamon, ground

Preparation:

Peel the banana and cut into chunks. Fill the measuring cup and reserve the rest. Set aside.

Wash the plums and cut each in half. Remove the pits and cut into small pieces. Set aside.

Wash the strawberries and remove the stems. Cut into bite-sized pieces and set aside.

Cut the cantaloupe in half. Scrape out the seeds and cut one large wedge. Peel and chop into small pieces and fill the measuring cup. Wrap the rest in a plastic foil and refrigerate for later.

Now, combine banana, plums, strawberries, and cantaloupe in a juicer and process until juiced. Transfer to a serving glass and stir in the cinnamon.

Add some crushed ice and serve immediately.

Nutrition information per serving: Kcal: 249, Protein: 4.8g, Carbs: 73.1g, Fats: 1.5g

49.   Black Grape Blueberry Juice

Ingredients:

1 cup fresh blackberries

1 cup black grapes, stems removed

1 cup fresh strawberries

1 medium-sized Fuji apple, cored

2 oz coconut water

Preparation:

Combine blackberries and strawberries in a colander. Wash under cold running water and set aside.

Rinse the grapes well and set aside.

Wash the apple and remove the core. Cut into bite-sized pieces and set aside.

Now, process blackberries, grapes, strawberries, and apple in a juicer. Transfer to serving glasses and stir in the coconut water.

Optionally, add some ice cubes before serving.

Nutritional information per serving: Kcal: 201, Protein: 4.3g, Carbs: 63.4g, Fats: 1.7g

50.   Strawberry Mint Juice

Ingredients:

1 cup frozen strawberries, chopped

1 cup fresh mint, torn

2 medium-sized red apples, cored

1 large honeydew melon wedge

2 oz coconut water

Preparation:

Chop the strawberries into halves or smaller pieces. Set aside.

Wash the mint thoroughly and torn with hands. Set aside.

Wash the apples and remove the core. Cut into bite-sized pieces. Set aside.

Cut the honeydew melon lengthwise in half. Scoop out the seeds using a spoon. Cut and peel 2 large wedges. Cut into small chunks and place in a bowl. Wrap the rest of the melon in a plastic foil and refrigerate.

Now, combine strawberries, mint, apple, and melon chops in a juicer. Process until juiced.

Transfer to serving glasses and stir in the coconut water.

Add ice cubes and serve immediately.

Nutritional information per serving: Kcal: 293, Protein: 4.5g, Carbs: 84g, Fats: 1.6g

51.   Salted Green Celery Juice

Ingredients:

1 cup fresh celery, chopped

1 cup fresh kale, chopped

3 large leeks, chopped

2 cups beet greens, trimmed

1 large cucumber

1 ginger knob, sliced

½ tsp Himalayan salt

Preparation:

In a large colander, combine celery, leek, beet greens, and kale. Rinse thoroughly under cold running water and drain. Chop all into small pieces and set aside.

Wash the cucumber and cut into thick slices. Set aside.

Peel the ginger and set aside.

Combine celery, leek, beet greens, kale, cucumber, and ginger in a juicer. Process until well juiced.

Transfer to serving glasses and stir in the salt.

Refrigerate for 10 minutes before serving.

Nutritional information per serving: Kcal: 230, Protein: 11.5g, Carbs: 63.2g, Fats: 2.1g

52.   Sweet Carrot Juice

Ingredients:

1 large carrot, sliced

1 cup apricots, pitted and halved

1 large lemon, peeled

1 medium-sized Granny Smith's apple, cored and chopped

1 tbsp agave nectar

2 oz water

Preparation:

Wash the apricots and cut in half. Remove the pits and fill the measuring cup. Reserve the rest for some other juice. Set aside.

Peel the lemon and cut lengthwise in half. Set aside.

Wash the carrot and cut into thick slices and set aside.

Wash the apple and remove the core. Cut into bite-sized pieces and set aside.

Now, combine apricots, lemon, carrot, and apple in a juicer and process until juiced.

Transfer to serving glasses and stir in the agave nectar and water.

Refrigerate for 15 minutes before serving.

Nutrition information per serving: Kcal: 243, Protein: 4.2g, Carbs: 69.3g, Fats: 1.3g

53.   Kiwi Avocado Juice

Ingredients:

2 kiwis, peeled

½ ripe avocado, peeled and sliced

1 large cucumber

1 cup frozen strawberries

1 small lime, peeled

2 tbsp fresh mint

Preparation:

Peel the kiwis and cut into halves, then into quarters. Set aside.

Peel the avocado and cut in half. Remove the pit and cut one half into thin slices. Reserve the other half in the refrigerator.

Wash the cucumber and chop into bite-sized pieces.

Wash the strawberries and cut into halves. Set aside.

Peel the lime and cut into quarters. Set aside.

Wash the mint leaves and soak in water for 10 minutes.

Process kiwis, cucumber, strawberries, lime, and mint in a juicer until nicely juiced.

Transfer to serving glasses and serve immediately.

Nutritional information per serving: Kcal: 181, Protein: 6.2g, Carbs: 41.9g, Fats: 21.9g

54.   Orange Cantaloupe Juice

Ingredients:

2 large oranges, peeled

1 cup cantaloupe, cubed

2 medium-sized radishes, trimmed

1 ginger root knob, 1-inch

1 tbsp liquid honey

½ cup pomegranate seeds

2 oz water

Preparation:

Peel the oranges and divide into wedges. Set aside.

Cut the cantaloupe in half. Scoop out the seeds and flesh. You will need about one large wedge for one cup. Cut and peel it. Chop into chunks and set aside. Reserve the rest of the cantaloupe in a refrigerator.

Wash the radishes and trim off the green parts. Cut into small pieces and set aside.

Peel the ginger root knob and set aside.

Cut the top of the pomegranate fruit using a sharp knife. Slice down to each of the white membranes inside of the fruit. Pop the seeds into a measuring cup and set aside.

Combine oranges, cantaloupe, radishes, ginger, and pomegranate seeds in a juicer and process until juiced. Transfer to serving glasses and stir in the honey and water.

Add few ice cubes or refrigerate for 10 minutes before serving.

Nutrition information per serving: Kcal: 279, Protein: 4.9g, Carbs: 82.3g, Fats: 0.8g

55.   Sweet Lemon Juice

Ingredients:

1 tbsp honey, raw

1 whole lemon, peeled

1 cup strawberries, chopped

1 whole lime, peeled

2 oz water

Preparation:

Peel the lemon and lime. Cut each fruit lengthwise in half and set aside.

Wash the strawberries and remove the stems. Cut into bite-sized pieces and set aside.

Now, combine lemon, lime, and strawberries in a juicer and process until juiced. Transfer to a serving glass and stir in the water and honey.

Refrigerate for 5 minutes before serving.

Enjoy!

Nutrition information per serving: Kcal: 81, Protein: 5.8g, Carbs: 20.8g, Fats: 1.4g

MEALS

Breakfast Recipes

1.   Salmon Pâté

Ingredients:

2 salmon fillets (1 inch thick), boneless and skinless

½ tsp of dry rosemary

1/8 tsp of sea salt

¼ tsp of chili pepper, ground

1 tbsp. of fresh lemon juice

Olive oil

Preparation:

Wash and pat dry the salmon fillets. Cut into bite size pieces and set aside. Heat up the olive oil in a large skillet and add the salmon pieces. Cook for about ten minutes stirring constantly. Remove from the heat and transfer to a food processor.

Add the remaining ingredients into the food processor. Process well until nicely combined. Serve with some fresh vegetables or whole wheat crackers of your choice.

Nutritional information per serving: Calories: 240, Protein: 20g, Carbs: 1.2g, Fats: 16g

2.   Detox Smoothie

Ingredients:

¼ cup of spinach, finely chopped

¼ cup of broccoli, finely chopped

1 tbsp. of walnuts, minced

1 tbsp. of hazelnuts, minced

2 cups of water

¼ tsp of ginger, ground

A handful of ice cubes

Preparation:

Combine the ingredients in a blender and blend for about 30 seconds. Serve cold.

Nutritional information per serving: Calories: 110, Protein: 17g, Carbs: 7g, Fats: 3g

3.   Avocado and Cashew Cream Purée

Ingredients:

2 whole eggs

2 egg whites

1 tbsp. of cashew butter

½ cup of skim milk

1 ripe avocado, roughly chopped

1 tbsp. of fresh mint leaves, finely chopped

A pinch of salt

Preparation:

Hard boil your eggs (about 10 minutes will be enough). Remove from the heat and allow it to cool.

Peel and cut the eggs. Mash with a fork. Separate the egg whites from yolks.

Peel and chop avocado. Place it in a blender. Add milk, eggs, egg whites, cashew butter, salt, and mint leaves.

Mix well for about 30 seconds. Serve cold.

Nutritional information per serving: Calories: 187, Protein: 12.8g, Carbs: 7g, Fats: 4.5g

4.   Fresh Tomato Smoothie

Ingredients:

1 cup of fresh tomato juice

2 small tomatoes, peeled

1 tbsp. of walnuts

1 tbsp. of honey

1 tbsp. of sesame seeds

Preparation:

Place the ingredients in a blender and blend for 20 seconds. Serve cold.

Nutritional information per serving: Calories: 111, Protein: 7g, Carbs: 27g, Fats: 1g

5.   Rice Pudding

Ingredients:

2 cups of skim milk (you can use almond milk for extra flavor)

½ cup of rice, precooked

1 tbsp. walnuts, finely chopped

1 tbsp. of hazelnuts, finely chopped

¼ tsp of salt

1 tsp of cinnamon, ground

½ tbsp. of sugar-free vanilla extract

Preparation:

In a medium sized saucepan bring 2 cups of milk to boil. Add the rice, nuts, salt, vanilla extract, and stir well. Cook for about 10 minutes, or until you get a creamy mixture. Stir in some cinnamon and remove from the heat. Allow it to cool in the refrigerator before serving.

Nutritional information per serving: Calories: 158, Protein: 14g, Carbs: 3g, Fats: 2g

6.   Smoked Salmon Spread

Ingredients:

1 cup of smoked salmon slices

½ cup of ground almonds

½ cup of fresh parsley

1 tsp of dry oregano

2 garlic cloves, crushed

2 tbsp. of olive oil

¼ cup of water

1/8 tsp of salt

Preparation:

Simply combine the ingredients in a food processor and mix well for about 30 seconds. Serve promptly with celery, or crackers, or side of choice.

Nutritional information per serving: Calories: 245, Protein: 41.3g, Carbs: 2g, Fats: 18g

7. Lean Lentil Burgers

Ingredients:

¾ cup of lentils, soaked

1 small red onion, peeled and finely chopped

½ medium-sized sweet potato, grated

1 small red pepper, finely chopped

2 slices of whole grain, buckwheat bread

2 tbsp. of rice flour

2 tbsp. bread crumbs

1 tsp. chia seeds

1 tsp of parsley, finely chopped

½ tsp of cayenne pepper

Salt and pepper to taste

Olive Oil

Other:

4 whole grain burger buns

1 medium-sized tomato, sliced

1 small onion, sliced

Several lettuce leaves

Preparation:

Heat up two tablespoons of olive oil over a large frying pan on medium heat. Add finely chopped onion and stir-fry until translucent. Add chopped pepper and continue to cook for a couple of more minutes, or until softened.

Remove from the heat and set aside.

Meanwhile, briefly cook the lentils (10 minutes should be enough). Drain and cool for a while.

Combine all fried ingredients with the lentils in a bowl and mix. Using your hands, shape 4 patties for the burgers.

Heat up 4 tablespoons of oil over a medium-high heat. Fry the burgers for 3-4 minutes on each side.

Serve with tomato, sliced onion, and lettuce. Add ketchup, or mustard, or mayo to your preference.

Nutritional information per serving: Calories: 294, Protein: 16.4g, Carbs: 59g, Fats: 6g

8. Mixed Berries Smoothie

Ingredients:

1 handful of mixed wild berries of your choice

1 tsp. of Stevia sweetener

1 tsp of ginger, minced

1 glass of water

Preparation:

Combine the ingredients in a blender and mix well for about 20 seconds. Serve cold.

Nutrition information per 1 serving: Calories: 19 Protein: 0.5g, Carbs: 7g, Fats: 0g

9.   Quick Coconut Cookies

Ingredients:

1 ½ cup coconut flour

1 cup rice flour

¾ cup of powdered stevia

3 eggs

6 tbsp. of honey (can be replaced with agave syrup)

2 tsp of baking powder

1 tsp of cinnamon

Preparation:

Preheat the oven to 300 degrees F. Place some baking paper over a baking sheet. Set aside.

Combine all dry ingredients in a large bowl. Gently whisk in the eggs, stevia, honey, and cinnamon. Mix well until smooth dough. Using your hands shape the cookies. Place on the baking sheet and bake for about 10-15 minutes.

Remove from the oven and allow it to cool for a while.

Nutrition information per 1 serving: Calories: 126 Protein: 1g, Carbs: 17g, Fats: 5.1g

10.　　Frozen Cherry Yogurt

Ingredients:

1 cup of cherry yogurt (can be replaced with vegan yogurt)

½ cup of fresh cherries

4 strawberries

2 tbsp. of honey

Preparation:

Combine the ingredients in a blender and mix well for 20 seconds. Pour in a glass and keep in the freezer for about 30 minutes. Serve cold.

Nutrition information per 1 serving: Calories: 110 Protein: 2g, Carbs: 21g, Fats: 1.5g

Lunch Recipes

11.   Cilantro Garlic Burgers

Ingredients:

2 cups of lentils, soaked

3 cloves of garlic, minced

½ cup of breadcrumbs (choose buckwheat bread)

¼ cup of Cheddar cheese (freshly grated is best, but whatever you have will work)

1 egg, beaten

2 cups of water

½ cup of rice flour

salt and pepper to taste

Preparation:

In a medium size bowl, mash lentils with folk then mix with garlic, breadcrumbs and cheddar cheese. Form into patties; set aside.

Whisk egg and water in a bowl and in another bowl mix the flour with a pinch of salt & pepper. Coat each patty gently with flour mixture, then dip into egg mixture bowl, then coat again with flour mixture. Heat olive oil over medium-high heat in a large skillet. Fry the burgers until lightly brown, about 2-3 minutes each side.

Serve on warm buckwheat bread or in a whole grain pita with cilantro, onion, tomatoes and whatever else you like – but this is optional.

Nutritional information per serving: Calories: 480, Protein: 38g, Carbs: 36g, Fats: 17g

12. Wild Salmon Salad with Rice

Ingredients:

7 oz. brown rice

5 oz. wild salmon fillet

4 tbsp. of extra virgin olive oil

5 oz. cherry tomatoes, halved

1 medium-sized onion, finely chopped

1 tbsp. of fresh mint, finely chopped

1 tsp of turmeric, ground

¼ tsp of sea salt

Preparation:

Place the rice in a deep pot. Add three cups of water and bring it to a boiling point. Cook for 15 minutes over medium heat, stirring occasionally. Remove from the heat and cool for a while.

Using a kitchen brush, spread the olive oil over the salmon fillet. Sprinkle with some salt and wrap tightly in aluminum foil. Add some more water in a pot and place the salmon in it. Bring it to a boil and cook for five minutes. Remove the salmon and unwrap. Chill for a while and cut into bite-size pieces.

In a large bowl, combine the salmon with rice, cherry tomatoes, chopped onion, mint, and turmeric.

Season with some more sea salt and olive oil, toss to combine and serve.

Nutritional information per serving: Calories: 171, Protein: 20g, Carbs: 17.8g, Fats: 6g

13.   Red Salmon Fillet

Ingredients:

1 pound of fresh salmon, sliced into 1 inch slices

½ cup of olive oil

1 tbsp. of garlic powder

½ tsp of sea salt

1 tbsp. of dry parsley

2 tbsp. of ground red pepper

1 small onion, chopped

1 lemon, sliced

Preparation:

Combine the olive oil, garlic powder, sea salt, dry parsley, and ground red pepper in a large bowl. Place the salmon slices in it, cover and marinate for about an hour.

Preheat the oven to 350 degrees F. Place the marinated salmon slices in a small baking dish. Bake in oven for 35 minutes. Remove from the oven, and serve with onions and lemon slices.

Nutritional information per serving: Calories: 240 Protein: 58g, Carbs: 0g, Fats: 17g

14.   Grilled Chicken Breast with Ginger Sauce

Ingredients:

4 oz. chicken meat, skinless and boneless

2 tbsp. olive oil

Preheat a non-stick grill pan over medium-high temperature. Cut the chicken meat into a bite size cubes. Add to the skillet and stir-fry with the olive oil for about 10 minutes.

Remove from the pan serve with ginger sauce.

How to prepare ginger sauce

Ingredients:

½ ounce of ginger root, peeled and chopped

1 garlic clove, crushed

1 tbsp. of fresh lemon juice

1 tsp of apple cider vinegar

¼ cup of chopped onion

Preparation:

Combine the ginger sauce ingredients in a blender and mix well for 20 seconds. Keep in the refrigerator for at least 20 minutes before serving.

Nutritional information per serving: Calories: 157 Protein: 30.8g, Carbs: 0g, Fats: 3.5g

15. Chilean Sea Bass Fillets

Ingredients:

4 oz. fresh sea bass fillets

1 lemon, sliced

¼ cup of lemon juice

1 tsp of dry rosemary, ground

1 tbsp. of fresh parsley, finely chopped

¼ tsp of pepper

Preparation:

Wash and clean the fish. Pat dry and cut in half.

Combine the lemon juice, dry rosemary, fresh parsley, and pepper in a large bowl. Soak the fish fillets with the bowl mix and leave in the refrigerator for 30 minutes to one hour.

Meanwhile, preheat the oven to 320 degrees F. Spread some baking sheets over a baking dish and set aside.

Remove the fish from the refrigerator and transfer to the baking sheet. Add some of the marinade on top of the fillets and bake for 30 minutes.

Remove from the oven, sprinkle with some more marinade and serve with lemon slices.

Nutritional information per serving: Calories: 77 Protein: 11.5g, Carbs: 0.2g, Fats: 3.5g

16. Crab Stew

Ingredients:

1 cup of diced tomatoes

4 oz. of frozen crab meat

1 tbsp. of dried basil

1 cup of fat free fish stock

1 cup of water

Pinch of pepper

1 oz. of tomato paste

3 celery stalks, washed, chopped

1 finely chopped onion

4 garlic cloves, crushed

Preparation:

Heat up a non-stick frying pan, to a medium temperature. Add chopped celery, onions, and about 2 tbsp. of water. Stir-fry for about 10 minutes. Remove from the heat and transfer to a deep pot. Add the remaining ingredients and cook for about 1 hour over a medium temperature.

Serve warm.

Nutritional information per serving: Calories: 177 Protein: 15g, Carbs: 4g, Fats: 0.5g

17.   Tomato Soup with Celery

Ingredients:

2 oz. tomato, peeled and roughly chopped

Pinch of pepper

1 celery stalk, washed and finely chopped

1 onion, diced

1 bay leaf

1 tbsp. of fresh basil, finely chopped

Fresh water

Preparation:

Preheat the non-stick frying pan over a medium-high temperature. Add the onions, celery, and fresh basil. Sprinkle some pepper and stir-fry for about 10 minutes, until caramelized.

Add the tomato and about ¼ cup of water. Reduce the heat to low and cook for about 15 minutes, until softened. Now add about 1 cup of water and bring it to a boil. Remove from the heat and serve with 1 bay leaf.

Nutritional information per serving: Calories: 21 Protein: 0.7g, Carbs: 4.9g, Fats: 0.9g

18. Grilled button mushrooms

Ingredients:

4 oz. button mushrooms

1 tsp fresh dill

½ tsp of garlic powder

Preparation:

Preheat a non-stick grill pan over a medium-high temperature. Clean, wash, and cut each mushroom in half. Grill for 5 minutes while stirring constantly. Remove the mushrooms from the heat and transfer to a serving platter. Sprinkle with some garlic powder and top with fresh dill. Serve warm.

Nutritional information per serving: Calories: 119 Protein: 22g, Carbs: 1.5g, Fats: 1.7g

19.   Mesclun Salad with Mussels

Ingredients:

4 oz. fresh mussels, de-bearded

1 onion, peeled and finely chopped

1 garlic clove, crushed

5 tbsp. of fresh lemon juice

¼ cup of fresh parsley, finely chopped

1 tbsp. of rosemary, finely chopped

1 oz. lettuce

1 oz. of arugula leaves

1 medium cherry tomato, for decoration

Sea salt to taste

Preparation:

Rinse and drain the mussels. Set aside.

Heat up a non-stick frying pan over medium-high temperature. Peel and finely chop the onion. Reduce the heat to medium temperature and add the chopped onion.

Add about ¼ cup of water. Stir-fry for several minutes, until crisp-tender. Now add the mussels and finely chopped parsley. Cook for about 20 minutes, stirring regularly. When all the water has evaporated, add garlic and chopped rosemary and stir well again.

In a large salad bowl, combine the mussels with arugula and lettuce. Add the lemon juice, sprinkle with some salt, and decorate with one cherry tomato. Serve promptly.

Nutritional information per serving: Calories: 78 Protein: 17g, Carbs: 6g, Fats: 9g

20.   Thai Mushrooms with Ginger

Ingredients:

1 cup of Gouda cheese, chopped into cubes

3 tbsp. of ginger sauce

1 tbsp. of extra virgin olive oil

2 tbsp. of fresh ginger, ground

2 cloves of garlic

2 tbsp. of minced fresh chili peppers

½ cup of fresh button mushrooms

1 cup of fresh yellow pepper, chopped

1 cup of green beans, cooked

2 tbsp. of teriyaki sauce

¼ cup of water

¼ cup of fresh basil, chopped

1 small onion, peeled and sliced

2 cups of brown rice, precooked

Preparation:

Combine the ingredients in a non-stick frying pan or a wok. Heat up the stove to a medium temperature and fry the ingredients for about 20 minutes, while stirring constantly.

Serve with brown rice.

Nutritional information per serving: Calories: 157 Protein: 30g, Carbs: 29g, Fats: 11.9g

Dinner Recipes

21.   Warm Quinoa and White Beans

Ingredients:

1 cup of quinoa, precooked

1 cup of white beans, precooked

3 tbsp. of hazelnuts, roasted

½ cup of fresh parsley

1 small onion, peeled and chopped

2 garlic cloves

¼ tsp of salt

5 tbsp. of extra virgin olive oil

1 cup of button mushrooms, sliced

¼ cup of cranberries, dry

Preparation:

Combine the hazelnuts, parsley, salt and 3 tbsp. of olive oil in a food processor. Blend well for 30 seconds. Heat up the remaining olive oil in a large skillet. Add chopped onion and garlic. Stir well and fry for several minutes, until nice golden color. Add cooked quinoa, white beans, button mushrooms, and mix well. Cook and stir for 5 more minutes, until the water evaporates. Remove from the heat and transfer to a large bowl. Add hazelnut blended mixture and ¼ cup of cranberries. Mix well and serve warm.

Nutritional information per serving: Calories: 189 Protein: 26.9g, Carbs: 39.6g, Fats: 8.9g

22.   Mediterranean Sea Bream

Ingredients:

2 pounds of fresh sea bream

½ cup of extra virgin olive oil

1 whole lemon, sliced

4 rosemary sprigs

1 tbsp. of dry mint, ground

3 garlic cloves, crushed

¼ tsp of red pepper

Salt to taste

Preparation:

Wash and clean the fish. Cut lengthwise and remove entrails. In a medium bowl, combine the olive oil with dry mint, crushed garlic cloves, and red pepper. Brush the fish with this mixture and stuff with lemon slices and rosemary sprigs.

Place 2 tablespoons of olive oil on a non-stick frying pan. Heat up the stove to a medium temperature and fry the fish for about 6 minutes on each side.

Nutritional information per serving: Calories: 117 Protein: 17g, Carbs: 0g, Fats: 7.5g

23.   Chicken Breast with Garlic and Parsley

Ingredients:

1 large chicken breast piece, skinless and boneless, cut into 1-inch-thick pieces

¼ cup of extra virgin olive oil

3 garlic cloves, crushed

½ cup of fresh parsley leaves

1 tbsp. of fresh lime juice

Salt to taste

Preparation:

In a medium bowl, combine the olive oil with crushed garlic cloves, finely chopped parsley, fresh lime juice and some salt (about ¼ tsp will be enough). Wash and pat dry the chicken meat and cut into 1-inch-thick pieces. Pour the olive oil mixture over the meat and let it stand for about 15 minutes.

Preheat the grill pan over a medium temperature. Add some marinade in the grill pan (about 2 tbsp.), then add the chicken fillets and cook for about 15 minutes while stirring occasionally.

Remove from the pan and serve with some vegetables of your choice.

Nutritional information per serving: Calories: 146 Protein: 33g, Carbs: 0g, Fats: 6.9g

24.   Oven Baked Veal with Sweet Cabbage

Ingredients:

8 oz. veal cutlets

17 oz. sweet cabbage, shredded

1 small onion, finely chopped

1 garlic clove, crushed

¾ cup of fresh tomato paste

1 medium-sized red pepper, sliced

½ tsp. salt

¼ tsp of ground black pepper

Olive oil

Preparation:

Preheat the oven to 350 degrees F. Spread some olive oil over a baking dish and place the cutlets in it. Bake for 20 minutes, or until lightly charred.

Meanwhile, heat up two tablespoons of olive oil in a large skillet on medium-high. Add the onion and crushed garlic. Stir-fry for 2-3 minutes, stirring constantly. Now add cabbage, sliced pepper, and fresh tomato paste. Cover and reduce the heat to medium-low. Cook for about 15 minutes. Remove from the heat and set aside.

Remove the cutlets from the oven and add cabbage mixture onto the cutlet baking dish. Season with some salt and ground black pepper. Cover the baking dish with aluminum foil and return to the oven. Bake for 30 minutes then serve.

Nutritional information per serving: Calories: 118, Protein: 8.7g, Carbs: 9.1g, Fats: 5.4g

25.   Sweet Potato and Peas Patties

Ingredients:

1 cup of green peas, cooked

1 sweet potato

½ cup of Parmesan cheese

½ cup of breadcrumbs

½ tsp. of salt

¼ tsp of freshly ground black pepper

1 egg

4 tbsp. of olive oil

Preparation:

Slice the sweet potato into one-inch-thick slices. Place in a deep pot and add enough water to cover. Bring it to a boil and cook until tender, for about 10-15 minutes. Remove from the heat, drain and allow to cool.

Transfer the cooked sweet potato slices to a food processor. Add green peas and process until smooth purée. Remove from the food processor and add salt, one egg, and black pepper. Mix well with a fork and using your hands, shape patties.

Heat up some olive oil in a medium-sized skillet. Roll each patty in breadcrumbs and fry for about three minutes on each side. Top with Parmesan cheese and serve.

Nutritional information per serving: Calories: 365, Protein: 12.4g, Carbs: 54.6, Fats: 14.1g

26.   Celery with Gorgonzola

Ingredients:

½ cup of celery, finely chopped

1 medium-sized pear, sliced

½ cup of toasted almonds

½ cup gorgonzola cheese, chopped

For the dressing:

1 medium-sized orange, juiced

3 tsp. of horseradish

2 tsp. of honey

1 garlic clove, crushed

½ tsp. salt

¼ tsp. ground pepper

2 tbsp. of olive oil

Preparation:

Combine the dressing ingredients in a glass jar with a tight lid. Lock the lid and shake well to combine. Set aside.

Place the sliced pear on a serving bowl. Add chopped celery, toasted almonds, and chopped gorgonzola. Toss to combine.

Drizzle with dressing and serve cold.

Nutritional information per serving: Calories: 302, Protein: 4.5g, Carbs: 21.3g, Fats: 19.8g

27.   Simple Lobster Recipe

Ingredients:

1 whole lobster

¼ cup of extra virgin olive oil

1 tbsp. of ground red pepper

½ tsp. of sea salt

¼ tsp. of black pepper

Preparation:

Preheat the oven to 350 degrees F. Meanwhile, combine the olive oil with sea salt, ground red pepper, and ground black pepper. Wash and cut the lobster in half along the long side. Place the lobster on a baking sheet and pour this mixture over it. Cook for about 10 minutes, until lightly golden color. Serve warm.

Nutritional information per serving: Calories: 111 Protein: 20g, Carbs: 0g, Fats: 6g

28.   Roasted Veggies with Grated Cheddar

Ingredients:

½ cup of beetroot, peeled and diced

½ cup of green beans, cooked and drained

½ cup of Brussel sprouts, chopped

½ cup of pumpkin, peeled and chopped

½ cup of carrot, chopped

1 cup of fresh tomatoes, roughly chopped

1 small onion, sliced

½ cup of cooked lentils

2 garlic cloves, minced

1 cup of finely chopped silver beet

Pinch of salt and pepper

3 tbsp. of olive oil

1 cup of grated Cheddar cheese

Preparation:

Preheat the oven to 350 degrees F. In a large bowl, combine beetroot, green beans, Brussel sprouts and pumpkin. Add 1 tbsp. of olive oil and some salt to taste. Place on an oven tray and bake for about 20 minutes.

Meanwhile, heat up the remaining oil in a medium sized saucepan. Add onions and carrot and fry for about 5 minutes, stirring constantly. Add diced tomatoes and chopped silver beet. Season with pepper and gently simmer for about 20 minutes.

In a large serving bowl, place the precooked lentil and top with the fried mixture. Serve the lentils topped with the roasted vegetables, and cheddar cheese.

Nutritional information per serving: Calories: 195 Protein: 32g, Carbs: 35g, Fats: 10.9g

29. Spinach Muffins

Ingredients:

1 ½ cup of buckwheat flour

½ cup of rice flour

1 tbsp. of baking powder

½ tsp of salt

1 cup of skim milk

2 eggs

¼ cup of olive oil

¼ cup of sour cream

¼ cup of spinach, cooked

Muffin molds

Preparation:

In a large bowl, combine all dry ingredients. Gently whisk in milk and crack 2 eggs. Mix very well, even with an electric mixer. This will give you a nice, smooth muffin dough. Now add spinach and sour cream into the dough and mix well again. Shape the muffins using muffin molds.

Preheat the oven to 300 degrees F. Bake muffins for about 20 minutes.

Nutritional information per serving: Calories: 174 Protein: 9g, Carbs: 21g, Fats: 7.8g

30.   Thai Trout

Ingredients:

1 pound of fresh trout

1 cup of fish stock

½ cup of olive oil

1 tbsp. of ground turmeric

½ cup of chopped celery

2 garlic cloves, crushed

2 tbsp. of fresh lime juice

¼ tsp of sea salt

1 cup of Thai vegetable mix, for serving

Preparation:

Wash and clean the trout. Pat dry and set aside.

In a deep pot, combine the fish stock with all the other ingredients. Bring it to boil and add the trout. Boil for about 10 minutes.

Meanwhile, heat up the grill pan over a medium temperature. Remove the fish from the pot and transfer to a grill pan. Add ¼ cup of fish stock in the pan and fry for several minutes.

Serve with Thai vegetable mix.

Nutritional information per serving: Calories: 287 Protein: 34g, Carbs: 9g, Fats: 12g

Salad Recipes

31.   Veal Salad with Fresh Veggies

Ingredients:

1 pound of veal cutlets

1 large tomato, chopped

1 large green pepper, chopped

½ cup of cabbage, grated

2 tbsp. of olive oil

Pinch of salt

Preparation:

Heat up the olive oil over medium temperature in a large frying pan. Fry the veal cutlets for about 10 minutes on each side. Remove the veal and cut further into bite size pieces and combine with the grated cabbage, green pepper, and chopped tomato in a large salad bowl. Add some salt to taste and serve.

Nutritional information per serving: Calories: 247 Protein: 44g, Carbs: 14g, Fats: 17g

32. Homemade Tuna Salad

Ingredients:

1 (12oz) tuna steak

¼ cup of spring onions, chopped

4 tbsp. of extra virgin olive oil

¼ tsp. of sea salt

¼ tsp. of chili pepper

1/8 tsp. of white pepper, ground

1 tbsp. of fresh lemon juice

Preparation:

Heat up two tablespoons of extra virgin olive oil over a medium-high temperature on a large skillet. Season the tuna steak with chili pepper, white pepper, and salt, and then place on skillet. Cook for 5 minutes on each side.

Remove from the skillet and cool for a while. Flake the tuna steak into small pieces and mix with spring onions in a large bowl. Top with two tablespoons of olive oil and sprinkle with fresh lemon juice. Serve warm or cold.

Nutritional information per serving: Calories: 212 Protein: 25g, Carbs: 14g, Fats: 11g

33.   Lettuce and Tomato Salad

Ingredients:

2 oz. tomato, roughly chopped

1 oz. lettuce, finely chopped

1 tsp. of apple cider vinegar

¼ tsp. of sea salt

½ tbsp. extra virgin olive oil

Preparation:

Place the chopped tomatoes and lettuce in a large salad bowl and toss. Season with salt, apple cider vinegar and olive oil, and then serve.

Nutritional information per serving: Calories: 19 Protein: 1g, Carbs: 7g, Fats: 7g

34.   Chicken Salad

Ingredients:

3 skinless, boneless chicken breast halves

1 cup of chopped lettuce

1 medium onion, peeled and sliced

5 cherry tomatoes

2 tbsp. of low fat sour cream

1 tbsp. of olive oil

1 tsp. of chopped parsley

1 tbsp. of extra virgin olive oil

1 tsp. of minced chili pepper

1 tbsp. of lemon juice

Pinch of salt to taste

Preparation:

Cut the chicken breast halves into small cubes. In a medium bowl, mix the olive oil, chopped parsley, minced chili pepper and lemon juice to make a marinade sauce. Put the chicken cubes on a baking sheet, sprinkle with marinade and bake at 350 degrees F for about 25 minutes. Remove from the oven. And let cool.

Meanwhile, in a large salad bowl, mix cherry tomatoes with chopped lettuce, sliced onion and low fat cream. Toss with chicken cubes, season with salt and olive oil and serve.

Nutritional information per serving: Calories: 187 Protein: 21.4g, Carbs: 7g, Fats: 2.5g

35.   Arugula Salad with Berries

Ingredients:

2 oz. fresh arugula

1 orange, peeled and sectioned

5 fresh strawberries, squared

¼ cup of fresh blueberries

1 tbsp. of honey

3 tbsp. of fresh lime juice

5 tbsp. of fresh orange juice

¼ tsp of ground cinnamon

Preparation:

In a small bowl, whisk together 1 tablespoon of honey with fresh lime juice, fresh orange juice, and ground cinnamon. In a large salad bowl, place the berries and strawberry squares and the arugula, then mix. Top the salad with the honey mixture and toss. Serve cold.

Nutritional information per serving: Calories: 72 Protein: 3g, Carbs: 19g, Fats: 3.7g

36.   Spring Onions Salad

Ingredients:

3 spring onions, finely chopped

¼ cup of sweet corn

1 tbsp. of fresh lime juice

2 tbsp. of olive oil

¼ tsp of salt

Preparation:

To prepare the onions you need to trim the roots away and strip off any extra outer leaves, then wash well. In a salad bowl, add two tablespoons of oil and place the chopped onions. Wait about 1 minute for the onions to absorb the oil and soften. Top with the sweet corn and mix together. Sprinkle with fresh lime juice and serve.

Nutritional information per serving: Calories: 122 Protein: 3.5g, Carbs: 21g, Fats: 7g

37.   Colorful Bean Salad

Ingredients:

1 cup of cooked beans of your choice

½ cup of sweet corn

3 spring onions, chopped

1 small red pepper, finely chopped

1 small green pepper, finely chopped

¼ tsp. of cilantro

½ tsp. of red wine vinegar

1 tsp. of fresh lemon juice

3 tbsp. of extra-virgin olive oil

A pinch of salt

Preparation:

In a small bowl, mix the olive oil with red wine vinegar, fresh lemon juice, cilantro, and a pinch of salt. In a large salad bowl, toss together the corn, cooked beans, and the peppers. Top with the olive oil mixture and serve.

Nutritional information per serving: Calories: 220 Protein: 24g, Carbs: 32g, Fats: 11g

38.   Baby Spinach Salad

Ingredients:

1 cup of cherry tomatoes

½ cup of Swiss cheese, cubed

1 cup of baby spinach

1 small orange, cubed

1 tbsp. of Parmesan cheese

1 tsp. of fresh lemon juice

Preparation:

Combine the ingredients in a large bowl and top with lemon juice. Mix well and serve.

Nutritional information per serving: Calories: 131 Protein: 20.5g, Carbs: 18g, Fats: 14g

39. Purple Salad

Ingredients:

1 piece of turkey breast, boneless and skinless

2 eggs

1 cup of red cabbage, grated

1 medium tomato, chopped

½ cup of olives

1 cup of scallions, chopped

½ cup sweet corn

4 tbsp. of olive oil

Pinch of salt

1 tbsp. of fresh lemon juice

Preparation:

Wash and pat dry the turkey meat then cut into 1-inch-thick strips. In a large skillet, heat up 2 tablespoons of olive oil on medium-high. Fry the turkey strips for about 10 minutes, turning them on all sides. Remove from the heat and transfer to a large salad bowl.

Meanwhile boil the eggs for about 7-8 minutes. Remove from the heat, drain and peel. Cut into slices.

Add the sliced eggs, chopped scallions, olives, chopped tomato, grated cabbage and sweet corn into the salad bowl with the fried turkey and mix well. Season with some salt and fresh lemon juice.

Nutritional information per serving: Calories: 186 Protein: 42g, Carbs: 38g, Fats: 17g

40. Sweet Corn and Tuna Salad

Ingredients:

2 cups of tuna, oil removed

½ cup of sweet corn

½ cup of red beans, precooked

1 small onion, chopped

¼ tsp of ground black pepper

¼ tsp of sea salt

1 tbsp. of olive oil

1 tbsp. of lemon juice

Preparation:

Peel and chop the onion into small pieces. Place the chopped onion in a salad bowl with the tuna and sweet corn. Add the precooked red beans and ground pepper and mix well. Season with olive oil, salt and lemon juice. Keep in the refrigerator for about 20-30 minutes before serving to serve cool.

Nutritional information per serving: Calories: 287 Protein: 31.7g, Carbs: 12.8g, Fats: 16g

Dessert Recipes

41.   Chocolate Cake with Strawberries

Ingredients:

2 cups of all-purpose flour

3 tsp. of baking powder

3 cups of milk

2 large bananas, mashed

2 cups of raw cocoa powder

5 tbsp. of agave syrup

3 tsp of vanilla extract

2 oz. fresh strawberries, chopped

Preparation:

Preheat oven to 350 degrees F. Use a small baking dish (8x8 inch) and place some baking paper in it.

Mix together all ingredients in a large bowl, except the strawberries. Add agave syrup, mashed bananas, and vanilla extract and slowly whisk in the milk. Mix well with an electric mixer. Now add the chopped strawberries and using a spoon mix again.

Pour the mixture evenly into your baking dish and bake for about 45 minutes. Remove from the oven and allow it to cool for a while before serving.

Nutritional information per serving: Calories: 487 Protein: 35g, Carbs: 45g, Fats: 24g

42.   Chocolate Brownies

Ingredients:

2 cups all-purpose flour

¼ cup of olive oil

½ cup brown sugar

1 cup of cocoa powder

1 large banana, mashed

2 tsp. baking powder

Preparation:

Mix all the ingredients in a large bowl using an electric mixer. Preheat the oven to 350 degrees F. Place some baking paper over a baking sheet. Bake for about 15 minutes, then cut into brownie square pieces and serve.

Nutritional information per serving: Calories: 243 Protein: 2.7g, Carbs: 39g, Fats: 10.1g

ADDITIONAL TITLES FROM THIS AUTHOR

70 Effective Meal Recipes to Prevent and Solve Being Overweight: Burn Fat Fast by Using Proper Dieting and Smart Nutrition

By Joe Correa CSN

48 Acne Solving Meal Recipes: The Fast and Natural Path to Fixing Your Acne Problems in Less Than 10 Days!

By Joe Correa CSN

41 Alzheimer's Preventing Meal Recipes: Reduce or Eliminate Your Alzheimer's Condition in 30 Days or Less!

By Joe Correa CSN

70 Effective Breast Cancer Meal Recipes: Prevent and Fight Breast Cancer with Smart Nutrition and Powerful Foods

By Joe Correa CSN

www.ingramcontent.com/pod-product-compliance
Lightning Source LLC
Chambersburg PA
CBHW030246030426
42336CB00009B/282